Battling Breast Cancer for Idiots

Battling Breast Cancer for Idiots

Billa Woollam

ISBN-13: 9781976150814
ISBN-10: 1976150817

Table of Contents

Introduction

This is a comprehensive guide to overcoming the physical and psychological changes associated with the recovery process and a survival tool for the aftermath of breast-cancer surgery.

My wish here is to instruct you on all sorts of things that may occur before and after your surgery, couched in a manner that includes a bit of humor, so you hopefully remember it more easily—a bit like that Super Bowl advertisement, which I thought was the best I'd ever seen. It was the one where you thought they were advertising a male performance-enhancing drug, when actually it was the little Italian motor car that looked like a pregnant roller skate, and I've never forgotten it. I started writing this partly to take my mind off the pain I was having when the drugs wore off—a bit like a Zen kind of thing (whoever Zen was). So in turn, I hope this does the same for you.

Hopefully this small instructive book will assist you in your speedy recovery with a few tips here and there on what you can expect and will be likely to experience. My ultimate goal is to one day become the J.K. Rowling of the self-help book.

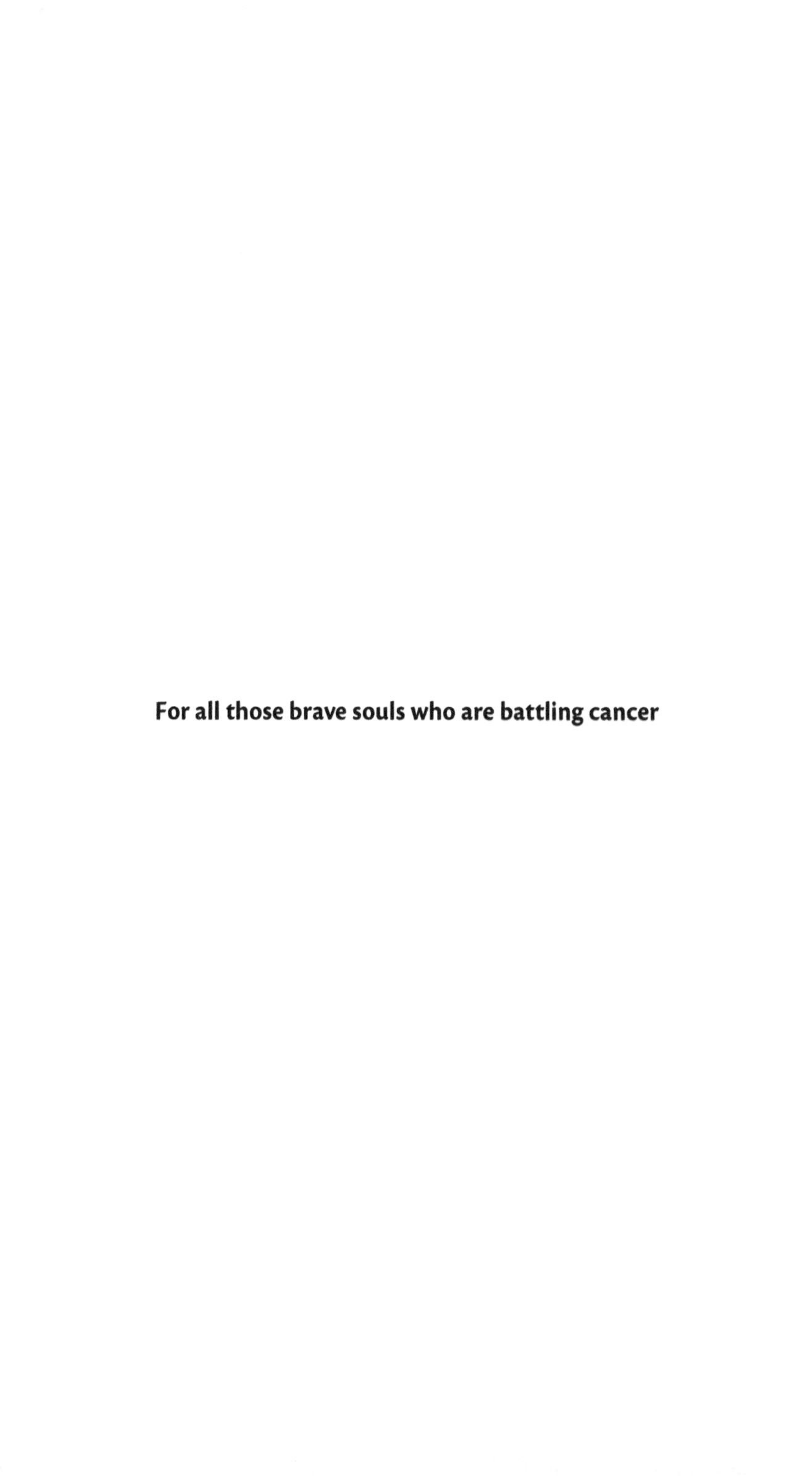

For all those brave souls who are battling cancer

Preface

ife is precious, as we all know. So in the preface to my book, I want to honor the memory of our dearest friend Patrick, who inspired us all with his love.

PATRICK JOSEPH COLLINS
October 20, 1959–January 28, 2013

This book is to honor the memory of our beloved friend Patrick Joseph Collins. He was a wonderful man from Cork in Ireland. He was one of the finest and most extraordinary human beings my husband, Richard, and I have ever met. He worked hard and played hard, and if we could all push as much into our lives and enjoy doing it as much as he did, the world would be a happier and gentler place.

He "shuffled off this mortal coil" at the age of fifty-three, and we were all shocked and upset that our beloved friend had passed. He made all our lives delightful, and as his family wrote in his obituary, "You came and made our lives beautiful. Memories of you remain captured in our hearts." He cherished his family and phoned them every single week, without fail, wherever he was in the world. He would call each member of his family separately every Saturday morning, bless his heart. Much to his friends' delight—and believe me, we are numerous—he lavished us all with fun, jokes, kindnesses, companionship; the list goes on and on. He made us aware of our own mortality and that we must enjoy every single moment on earth as it could be our last. He showed us all, by being the wonderful person he was, the most important priorities in life, and I don't need to remind any of you what they are. Pat was just meant to be in our lives, and we were the lucky recipients of his love.

We remember him visiting us in Houston the Christmas before he left this life. We had been out for a meal and had one or maybe two glasses of vino at most, as we exercise a lot of restraint. Anyway, I was doing the driving back home, and when we got into the house, neither Richard nor Pat was able to negotiate the alarm quickly enough. Of course, the police turned up about ten minutes later and—typical Pat—he followed me to the front door and said, "Would you like a glass of wine, officer?" Luckily they know us around the estate as "those Brits" and have been to our house a few times—just for the security thing, of course.

We all met around twenty-five years ago. We worked for a large British oil company and were posted in Alaska as expats. My husband and I both worked for this company in England at their research center just outside of London, and we left for Alaska in 1990. Richard is a corrosion engineer, Pat was a petroleum engineer, and I was a secretary, or administrative assistant, as they are now known.

We enjoyed our first Christmas in Alaska in 1990, and the following year, we were invited to Patrick's for Christmas. A few of the expats without children—not that Pat disliked children, far from it—were invited to his house for Christmas Day. It was our second Christmas Day in Alaska, and it was snowing, which was lovely. Richard and I were invited in, and I had a good old look around because, as my nephew rightly observed from a very young age, "You and mam (my sister, Barbara) are the nosiest women I know." I noticed lots of red wine already sitting open on the dining-room table. I asked Pat why, and like the gentleman he always was, he said, "The wine has to breathe, lass." I didn't know that twenty-five years ago, yet he never embarrassed me but forgave my ignorance, bless him.

Again on the topic of wine, later on in the evening someone spilled a glass of red over the beautiful new sweater my sister had just knit for me; she's a fabulous knitter. I did know that if you pour white on red, it's supposed to bring the stain out. So I asked Pat for a glass of white, and he said, "Do you want dry or sweet?" Every year for Christmas, we all received a box of books from Amazon. We would always say, "Ooh, it's our present from Pat." Pat's glass was always half full, usually with a very good wine.

Pat's house was on the hillside in Anchorage in the Chugach range of mountains, overlooking Anchorage and the whole of the Pacific Rim. You could see Denali and Mount Redoubt (which is an active volcano) to name only some of them, and as you can imagine, the view was spectacular.

Christmas at Pat's was bitterly cold, of course. Another of our friends was there too, Mike Webster, who is a petrophysicist for the same oil company. Mike is a Scot, and apart from his day job, he also plays the Scottish bagpipes. I have always loved the haunting sound of a single piper playing a Scottish lament, and I asked Mike if he would bring his pipes with him and play a lament for me outside later on in the evening. Not only did he agree to do this, but he dressed in the kilt and all the other accoutrements of the traditional Scottish piper. He stood there and played the lament outside, and the sound made the hair stand up on the back of my neck. This was a moment of magic for me and one I will never forget. The other people who lived up there must have heard Mike playing, and they would have had a magical and ethereal experience too.

One of our fondest and most special memories was our tradition at Christmas at our house. Richard and I used to have huge Christmas celebrations. They would span at least three days. Don't forget that this was at least twenty years ago. Sometimes there would be as many as twenty-five folk around the table. One Christmas, one of our friends couldn't join us, as he was on a foreign posting. Someone had a phone, and we all sang "Feliz Navidad" to him, which we'll never forget.

We started a lovely tradition around then, where I used to bring in the pudding after having served enough food to feed an army, and by then, it was getting on for bedtime. We would turn all the lights out, and Richard would set fire to the pudding, having doused it in brandy, and the blue flame was gorgeous. Pat would stand there at the same time and read from Dickens's *A Christmas Carol*, the passage where Mrs. Cratchit brings the pudding out of the copper. By the time Pat got up to perform, he was somewhat affected by "the lateness of the hour." Pat was the last person to read from that little book, and it's still in our dining-room sideboard with the page marked. It will always be there, never to be read again. Luckily, we have another copy.

So Pat, as you well know, we all loved you, and we miss you more than words can say. Even though you're not actually with us physically, I have a sneaking suspicion where I think you might be. The chap who played the part of Tony Soprano, the actor James

Gandolfini, died at the same age as Pat—fifty-three. He was once interviewed and asked what he thought Saint Peter would say to him when he arrived at the pearly gates. His response was, "Take over; I'll be right back." I'm sure Saint Peter gave the same retort to Pat on his arrival.

Credits

I want to thank my dearest friend, Linda Lillmars, in Alaska, for planting this germ of an idea…or was it a cockroach? Anyway, she asked why didn't I keep a journal day to day, noting changes in my recovery, how I was feeling, and so on, which gave me a few ideas. Over the next couple of days, I never stopped scribbling, making notes in a journal that I found by chance on the top of the washer. On the front cover were the words "Yesterday is history, tomorrow is mystery, today is a gift" (E. Roosevelt). I looked up at the ceiling and said, "Thank you," and picked it up, and one thing led to another.

After I received huge numbers of cards and flowers—which told me that my loved ones were thinking of me in my time of need—I told my husband that I was deeply touched and slightly overwhelmed by this. I said that I didn't think people liked me that much. He said, "They don't." My husband was sitting next to me while I was scribbling in this new journal, and it slowly occurred to me that he was secretly delighted that I was doing this instead of talking to him.

Diagnosis

was diagnosed with stage I breast cancer in November 2015. I went to Methodist West hospital on I-10 for my mammogram, as they had just opened their new Breast Care Center, and state-of-the-art technology was now available there. They took great care of me and caught my cancer very early. So do have a yearly mammogram because it's hugely important.

Telling your friends the news about your diagnosis

My friend Bobbie Bianchi in Alaska called me and said, "It's amazing the lengths that people will go to, to get attention." When we lived in Anchorage, I used to work with all these really talented people at a wonderful gallery called Artique Ltd., and we've been friends ever since.

Unbelievably, three days later, another friend, the artist and gallery manager, Susan Pennewell-Ellis, called me and told me that Bobbie was in the hospital for quadruple-bypass heart surgery.

Once I knew that she was out of the ICU and back in an ordinary room, safe and still with us, and sort of feeling a little more compos mentis (for Bobbie, anyway), I called her in her hospital room. When she answered, I simply said, "It's amazing the lengths that people..." Revenge is sweet.

I suddenly had to come to terms with the fact that I had cancer, and I needed to figure out what I was going to do to help myself. I talked to a few people apart from my doctors, of course. My sister told me about a theory called "mindfulness." Basically, if you concentrate on staring or looking intently at something, sort of like meditating, it takes your mind off the pain, hopefully. Well, I did just that. I lay down on the floor next to my dog, Sky, who is a yellow lab with a shiny black nose. I looked at her face for a good hour, but unfortunately the only thing that happened was that Sky just sniffed me a lot, and her breath wasn't too special either.

Our dear friends Dan and Amy Replogle sent me a great self-help book, which I started to read and really tried to persevere with, but unfortunately my concentration was shot, and I couldn't take it in. There are some really great and comprehensive self-help books out there, but please read them *before* your surgery. After surgery, forget it.

The University of Texas MD Anderson Cancer Center Team Appointments

Next, it was time to meet my team of doctors. They all looked like twenty-year-olds in their nice white doctor coats. When I saw them again in their scrubs just before I was taken down for my surgery, they looked about fifteen.

Plastic Surgeon
Before the procedure

My appointment with the plastic surgeon was scheduled next. Surprisingly, he drew on my breasts with a Sharpie. My husband Richard, who was observing from the back of the room, asked, "Are you planning on doing a spot of landscape gardening?"

The plastic surgeon then took several photos of me from the neck down, I suppose as a "before" for his "after" comparison. He assured me that the photos would not end up on social media, and I gave a sigh of relief. If they did happen to be published by mistake, I could always say that there was no proof that it was me.

Next, the surgeon asked me if I would like a breast reduction, because, he said, he was there anyway, and why didn't he do a two-for-one deal? I thought I'd just won the lottery, and I couldn't believe that this would be an option. I asked if it was covered by my insurance. When he said yes, I thought it was the best news I'd heard since the Dow Jones recovery. I agreed to this procedure, and I was smiling like a Cheshire cat. Richard said that he'd never seen anyone actually look forward to breast surgery before.

Next, the surgeon asked, "What size would you like to be?" I thought back and back and admitted that I used to be a 36B. He asked my size now, and I told him I was a 44DD. I said, "A 38B might be nice." He took a long, hard look at me and told me that he could just about manage a 38C, but a B was out of the question.

So the plan was set; the surgeon was going to give me a nice new pair of Barbie dolls, pointing, for once, in the same direction. Things were looking up, literally. Richard tried not to look disappointed when I agreed to have it done.

I remembered that I even had large breasts when I was ten years old. I was in the Brownies then, and unlike the other kids, I could never put anything at all in the top pockets of my uniform, as they were already full.

Come to think of it, this was 1963, only eighteen years after the end of the Second World War. Our uniforms were little brown cotton dresses, buttoned up to the neck, complete with a brown beret and a large brown leather belt. We all looked like the "Hitler Youth"...not terribly attractive. Our girl guide uniforms were even uglier. We all looked as though we were about to invade Poland!

Problems associated with large breasts prior to the procedure

I knew, with heightened self-knowledge, that having larger breasts made it difficult for my surgeons to find where they needed to be in order to work on me. I could only compare this to...perhaps a giraffe with a sore throat.

I attended a wedding, and I thought I had a suitable dress that might look reasonably OK on me. The dress was bright green with matching accessories. A child approached me, and I sensed that he had something he wanted to say. He told me that I looked like the Incredible Hulk.

Prior to my breast reduction, I tripped over the dog in the dark because the light bulb outside needed replacing. I fell face-down on the concrete, but my breasts hit the ground first, thereby saving my teeth. I told this "friend" of mine, who told her husband, who is the rudest, nastiest moron I have ever met in my entire life. Unbelievably, she told me what he'd said: "How was the concrete?"

Preparing for the Hospital
What to take with you and wear on the morning of your surgery

Your team will instruct you on suitable attire and give you a detailed list of items you will need for the procedure.

A shirt that opens at the front.

A bra that opens at the front.

Nothing else, as not everybody's honest.

What I did

I looked in my closet two days prior to surgery for a shirt. I hate myself in shirts, because large-breasted women really shouldn't wear button-down shirts at all. They not only look awful but also gape at the very place where they're not supposed to. This means that now you have to put a big safety pin in the middle, between the buttons, for it to look anywhere decent. So I went into my closet and found the only shirt of this type that I possessed: a big button-down shirt in blue linen that I bought five or six years ago. I brushed the dust off the shoulders, as it had been hanging there a good while, not having been worn. I reluctantly tried it on, and, of course, it still looked as bad—if not worse—than it did five or six years ago, the last time I tried it on.

"But," I thought, "maybe if I put on a nice scarf, or maybe a necklace with it, it might not look too bad." So I went back to my closet to try to find an accessory that would disguise my figure, and I saw this scarf hanging—one that I normally wouldn't look at twice. I draped it and thought, "That will be fine, as long as I don't forget my earrings and gray trousers, with some nice gray slingbacks to match." Who does that?

I arrived with my carefully chosen shirt and accessories, only to be shown into a room where I was immediately instructed to take them all off again.

Treatment

Postsurgery

I was wheeled into the recovery area, but of course, I was unaware and blissfully asleep, since I'd had four or five hours of anesthetic. Then I was wheeled into my own personal room, which could have been on Mars for all I knew. I woke up hours later and immediately winged off an e-mail to my loved ones, assuring them that I was still alive. This was a really bad idea, as I wasn't myself and not in control, to put it mildly.

Everyone noticed that I'd just come around from the anesthetic.

Oncologist

At the first postsurgery appointment with the oncologist, I was told that because of my diagnosis and as a result of the laboratory report on my tumor, I would not need to have chemotherapy, but I would need to have radiation. This was scheduled a few weeks after my surgery.

Initial consultation appointment

At my first appointment, on the very same day that the weather people issued a tornado warning for Houston, I experienced a panic attack in his office. By the time I calmed down enough to be coherent so that the doctor could talk to me, he asked if I was experiencing any memory loss. I said, "Yes, my short-term memory is not good...what was your question?"

Also, at this initial appointment, they asked about my family health history, which set the alarm bells ringing for me. After listing a catalog of family members' ailments and the causes of their demise for both sides of my family, I realized that I had inherited really bad genes.

I confessed that my uncle on my paternal side was a raging alcoholic. This amused Richard; he laughed out loud and said that he was tired of counting the number of skeletons emerging from my closet.

Radiation Oncologist

Next, I had my radiation appointment, where they explained in detail all the procedures I could expect. The doctor told me about my simulation, which was a kind of dress rehearsal for my radiation appointments. She told me that at the simulation, they would make a special mold of my body to be used at every session. This would be made specifically for me and would be stored in the radiation room with my medical number on it. The doctor then left the room, and they showed my husband, Richard, and me a video that explained what was going to happen.

At one point, they told me that they were going to give me a tattoo, a sort of x-marks-the-spot, where they'd concentrate the radiation on me. Richard was worried that the tattoo would be a rampant serpent.

We were still in the office watching the video when they told me, "Not to worry—you won't be radioactive." Richard was relieved that I wasn't going to glow green in the dark.

The date for my first radiation appointment was set. I didn't know if I'd be able to drive to my appointments every day, so I thought it was a sterling idea to use my new tricycle to get there. I hadn't used my tricycle in a while because I was recovering from my second hip replacement exactly one year ago and had not yet ventured out on it again. Richard was very skeptical about this idea, as the route was a very busy road on which there were no foot-paths, and I couldn't ride in the road; I was too wide (on the bike, of course).

Then I remembered that the doctors had told me that walking would be good exercise, because for the moment, I'd stopped lifting weights. So I asked Richard to clock the distance from our house to MD Anderson, thinking it couldn't be more than a couple of miles in one direction. He told me it was exactly six miles in one direction! Back to the drawing board.

Recovery

Anesthesia and the Inevitable Aftereffects Confusion

My team advised me that because of my procedure and its psychological effects, it was probably a good idea to seek the advice of a professional counselor. I assured the team that I'd already organized this because I was seeing one prior to my diagnosis anyway for other issues. So now I could go back to the same person, as she was familiar with how my brain worked.

Missed counselor appointments

My counselor left a message on my cell phone to tell me that I'd missed an appointment that I made prior to my surgery. She was not able to reach me on that phone, so then she called me on the house phone to leave the same message. I answered this call, thinking that she'd called me to see how I was. Because I hadn't heard my previous message on my cell or even been able to find it, I talked to her endlessly, and the poor soul couldn't get a word in. Finally, she had to interrupt to tell me that after talking to me for around forty-five minutes, she was late for a lunch engagement. She'd call me later.

I managed to find my cell phone and listened to her first message, which told me that I'd missed an appointment. Then I wanted to call her to apologize for missing the appointment, but I couldn't find her number.

Innocence

I have always been very naïve, and I believe most things people say to me; it's a bit sad, really. I'm definitely not the sharpest knife in the drawer either, so the two combined, together with the effects of anesthesia and heavy-duty painkillers, made me completely "lose the plot," and I went quite bonkers—for only a short time, of course. I had, at best, a very tenuous grip on reality.

Richard told me that the word "gullible" was no longer included in the *Oxford English Dictionary*. This worried me, to the point where I flicked through the *OED* and looked through the G section for the word. Richard simply said, "I rest my case."

Uncomfortable silences

Sometimes, people find it hard to know what to say or do when you're either in the hospital or going through major trauma, and there can be an uncomfortable silence. So someone should probably try to change the subject. My nephew Ben, who is a very kind and thoughtful chap, gets very uncomfortable if someone isn't happy, bless his heart. Even when he was a little boy, he would try to change the subject if someone got upset.

Once, years ago, my mam, Ben (who was around eight years old), an old school friend of my mam, and I were in our village pub for lunch in the North of England. We touched on a sensitive subject, and her friend burst into tears. There was a longish silence, and I could see that Ben was worried. After a few minutes had elapsed, he suddenly said, "Hands up—who likes Elvis Presley?" Of course, we all laughed, and I asked what on earth this had to do with anything. Ben said, "I just wanted to know, Auntie." So again, my Ben tried to help and save the day.

The negative aspects of recovery

I was talking at length to Richard about negative things that wouldn't help my long-term recovery. To change the subject, he said, "How about those Astros?"

Later, I was complaining bitterly to him at length that someone had upset me. He said, "How about those Rockets?"

I was talking way too much to a friend and getting overly excited about nothing. Richard did a hand signal, which we'd already agreed on, to shut me up and calm me down. He did this signal from the other side of the room, and I got the message loud and clear.

Forgetfulness and the home routine

I went to retrieve something from the laundry, which was supposed to be in our bathroom, but since leaving our bedroom to go to the laundry room, I'd forgotten what I was going in there for. By now Richard, who was aware of what was going on with me, simply shouted, "Bath mats!"

I was in our bathroom another time and asked Richard to unblock the "hers" sink, because it was clogged. I set about taking all my makeup out of the cupboard under the sink so he could get at the u-bend. I asked him to please hurry because I needed to use my sink. He simply asked, "How many sinks are in there?"

I got new painkillers that were really strong and needed to be taken with food and copious amounts of water. I said that I couldn't take the tablet until dinnertime, which was five hours away. Richard said, "You can have it with a snack at any time, with the copious amounts of water."

I was standing in our living room, naked and fresh out of the shower, while Richard helped me with my dressings. I was eternally grateful that the gardeners weren't outside.

I talked at length to the gentleman who looks after our pool, and forgot that he had a job to do.

Richard asked me if I liked a particular film on the TV and what I would like to watch. I told him that he could watch whatever he wanted, because I couldn't concentrate on following the dialogue anyway. So he went back to his NFL game. I was surprised that I was actually enjoying watching football and forgot that I didn't like it in the first place.

Technological issues

I tried to log on to my MD Anderson website, trying to pretend that I was great on the computer. I needed to do this because I'd been dragged, screaming, into the twenty-first century by Richard, who was only trying to help. He set up the whole thing for me—the password and everything—such that a donkey could log on.

He was still in bed, and I tried to log on because I wanted to show off and impress him. But I couldn't remember anything he'd set up for me, so...need I say more?

He woke up, finally, and once again helped me get onto the website. Now that I was in there, I scrolled through my list of future appointments and saw that I had one for pain management down-town at the medical center. I read the doctor's name, and because his name was listed surname first, in ordinary (not bold) font, for a brief and fleeting moment, I thought his name was "Billy the Kid.'"

Follow-Up Appointments

My first follow-up with the plastic surgery team arrived at my next appointment, hoping that I appeared as though I was behaving in a more lucid way than I was at the last appointment. That time, my doctor seemed a little concerned about my general state of mind, understandably. It was the same day that there was an accident downtown on a tall building, when the window cleaners' hanging basket collapsed on one side, and they had to be rescued.

We were shown into one of the doctor's consulting rooms, which, it has to be said, was rather small when filled with me, Richard, the doctor, his nurse, and a new doctor whom I hadn't met before. They were examining me when there was a clatter at the window; I looked around, and yes, the window cleaner was there in his basket, cleaning my personal window. I was being examined at that very moment, and I was relieved beyond sanity that the windows to the room were of obscure glass. Otherwise, the window cleaner would have witnessed something he'd rather forget.

Radiation and Its Side Effects
Hearing

I noticed a marked difference in my hearing, postradiation. Actually, it wasn't too good before my surgery, but of course I couldn't remember that. Anyway, we attended a work function, where there was a lot of background noise. Across the room, I spotted the wife of one of Richard's colleagues, who was recovering from major surgery herself. I went over to pay my respects and asked her how she was doing. She has a pronounced Boston accent and said she was recovering nicely from her heart transplant. I took a lock of her hair, touched it, and then told her, "Wow, yes, it does look great. Is it a Bosley?"

Constipation

I was very concerned when I realized that I hadn't been to the toilet in about three days. So I dialed my doctor's number, or so I thought, and left a very detailed, graphic message about it and then asked if he could please call me back. I had in fact dialed Richard's work number while his speaker phone was on in a meeting.

The increased growth of facial hair

I noticed that I appeared to be growing a lot more facial hair. My nephew noticed this and politely asked me if I was trying to grow a beard.

Lack of appetite and the positive attitude with regard to inevitable weight loss

When I first joined Weight Watchers decades ago, everything was handwritten. Over the years, they've changed things numerous times, and now they're in the space age with websites and twenty-first-century technology.

This was a source of irritation for me over the years, as every time I rejoined with a new determination and vigor and the knowledge that "this time it's going to work," they'd changed to a completely different program. Now I didn't need to rejoin again. Finally, with a sigh of relief, I could throw out all the cookbooks, points calculators, and plastic spoon measures, the accumulation of which spanned a quarter of a century.

Years ago—maybe fifteen or so—extra treats in my diet in addition to my daily food allowance were referred to as "floaters," which is also a British colloquialism for human waste. Weight Watchers gave me a plastic graph to put on the fridge to keep track of my calories, floaters, and the like. Imagine my surprise when Richard saw this and left me the following message on my graph: "Eat s**t—fifty million flies can't be wrong."

I could now buy really cheap bras from Walmart that fastened in the front and were surprisingly comfortable. I no longer had to wear the sort that involved the design skills of a civil engineer.

Someone told me that their large-breed dog had gained forty-five pounds in six months, and no longer did I have to empathize and say, "I know how he feels."

Rehabilitation after Surgery
Light chores in the home

I worked with a lot of very witty people at the research center, some of whom, because they were so clever, were quite odd and a little eccentric. This one friend of ours once told me, "The greatest test for an army cook is the ability to make a profiterole under fire!" So, ladies and gentlemen, a few more pointers.

It's a good idea to try to get back to normal as soon as you can, to make yourself feel involved in the home again—but do take it easy. Day by day, gradually, you will reap the benefits of performing your normal household tasks. A little light cooking can be very beneficial and will give you a greater sense of usefulness each day of your recovery.

Cooking

My first foray into the kitchen, however, didn't go as smoothly as I would have liked. I decided to cook a ready-made dinner that I bought prior to my surgery in case I didn't feel like cooking. I bought it from one of the big-box stores, cooked it straight from my freezer, and presented it to Richard, trying to please him and thinking that I was doing a great job. It was an Asian rice dish, and I was supposed to add some chicken to go with it. Of course I forgot and served it to him without the chicken. He looked first at the food and then at me and said, "Isn't there something that should go with this?" I realized that, yes, he was right—but he still ate it anyway. He didn't want to upset me because I wasn't very well.

I cooked another meal, hoping for an improvement over the first attempt. I tried really hard and hoped that this time I'd have a culinary success. Simultaneously, we both took a few bites. Richard looked at me and said, "This is genuinely disgusting." He was right about this one, too.

Making a cup of tea

I made myself a cup of tea, and of course I forgot about it. I found my cup of tea around half an hour later, and it was cold. So my intention was to reheat it in the microwave. Instead, I put it in the fridge, thereby making it slightly colder than it was before.

Making a cocktail

I asked Richard if he'd like a cocktail, seeing as it was New Year's Eve. He asked for a rum and Coke. I had Captain Morgan's rum, but no Coke. So I said, "I have the rum, but no Coke. How about a Dr. Martin?"

Looking after pets

Pets are very sensitive, as we all know. My dog, Sky, knew that there was something not quite the ticket with her mam…well, perhaps a little more so than normal. She followed me around the house all day to make sure I was OK, bless her. I'm sure she could smell the difference in me!

I petted Sky, and instead of saying, "Give me a love," I said, "Give me a call."

Sky was hovering around her water bowl. She's an old lady, and sometimes I'm confused as to whether she wants to go out or she wants me to top up her water. So I said, "Do you want to go out, baby, or do you want a glass of wine?"

Friends and social contact

We had arranged a party at our house long before I was diagnosed. We still went ahead with the party, two weeks after my surgery, because I said our friends would cheer me up and take my mind off what had happened to me.

I was delighted that I'd bought a nice new beaded caftan to wear prior to diagnosis, which I now knew would hide my drains.

I then danced at said party—one dance only—with worried friends looking on, trying not to say anything.

The music was rock 'n' roll, because I'm in my sixties. I decided that it was a good idea to dance with a partner, Jim House, and he twirled me, which I'd always enjoyed prior to surgery. When they removed my tumor, they had also removed my lymph nodes under my left arm. This made it painful to raise my arm. Jim didn't know this of course, so guess which arm he twirled me on?

Richard shouted at my partner for twirling me because of my lymph nodes.

My first shopping trip

I now felt confident enough to venture out on my first grocery-shopping trip. Richard drove me there, as I really shouldn't have been on the road yet, for the sake of the other drivers as much as anything. He took me to my nearest store, and I really enjoyed this new feeling of independence and freedom. I savored everything in a fresh, new way. I was delighted that the bread was arranged in an interesting way, that they seemed to have a huge variety of sausages available, and so on. Now, I was in the seasonal aisle admiring a big red plastic heart to hold chocolates, as it was nearly Valentine's Day. I saw Richard approaching me with a slightly irritated look on his face.

He asked me if I was done yet, as it had already been over an hour. I told him I was nearly finished, and to divert his attention, I asked him to go and choose his favorite ice cream. He chose his flavors, and we were on our way to the checkout when I realized that there was no line at the customer-service desk, and it was the day of the record lottery payout. So I wandered off to get a lottery ticket.

He pulled me back to reality and said, quite rightly, that we had to pay for our groceries first.

So we went to the checkout, and I was amazed at myself for how logically I was putting our groceries on the conveyor belt. It's the first time in my life that I'd actually put all the frozen stuff there first, then the veggies, then the cans, and then the rest of it. Richard was getting more irritated by the minute, as the time lapse was now around an hour and a half. Finally, we paid and were headed for the car when Richard reminded me, "Now you can get the lottery ticket."

So I went back in the store to the customer-service desk. The person in front of me there was doing a money order, and it took about thirty minutes to do the transaction. Back at the car, I thanked Richard for patiently waiting for me for around two hours in total. He said, "I said take your time, not a vacation!" Of course, I didn't win the lottery, *again*

Exercising

Another great way to get a bit of normality into your recovery process is to start lightly exercising again. I must tell you how important it is to take it very easy. First, start by gently walking around the house, then to the mailbox, and so on, until you start to feel stronger again. As soon as you feel a bit stronger, you can think about doing a bit of training or exercising at the gym.

Dancing

I was in the kitchen trying to create culinary miracles, and I heard my favorite Def Leppard track on the radio. I'd always loved dancing—especially while cooking. I started to dance, while stirring the pot on the stove at the same time. Richard came in and definitely thought I'd "lost the plot." This was just the sort of thing I should have been doing postsurgery and in my sixties.

Psychological Differences, Postsurgery Euphoria and heightened appreciation

I experienced an intense feeling I have never had before: a heightened appreciation for everyday things that would have brought me pleasure anyway but were now magnified several times over. It doesn't take a lot to please me anyway; even a new pattern on a box of tissues delights me. I sensed an eagerness to do things that I previously probably would not have even thought about or attempted. I'm a relatively spontaneous person, generally speaking, but now this is me magnified several times, if you can imagine anything worse.

Joie de vivre and exhilaration

I felt so great and happy about most things and most people. I could only compare this great feeling to that of Ebenezer Scrooge when he woke up on Christmas morning.

Breast-cancer walk

I registered for a thirty-nine-mile walk downtown in Houston, two days after I got home from surgery. I was assured by my friends that they would be my "team" and walk with me...until I told them how long it was. I agreed that, yes, a three-mile walk might be more appropriate, but I was going to do the thirty-nine-mile one anyway.

I received a call from my very own personal walking coach. She was a very nice and encouraging lady, but in the course of the conversation, she told me that at the halfway point on the walk—which spanned a couple of days—I would get to stay overnight in a tent with a complete stranger. I told her that unless she arranged a hotel room for me, complete with running water and clean sheets, all to myself, I wouldn't even consider doing it.

Then she sent me all the blurbs associated with the walk in the mail, and I couldn't concentrate enough to read the details anyway.

I realized that my eagerness to register was perhaps a little, shall we say, overambitious.

Worst-Case Scenario Preparations
Plans for an uncertain medical outcome

I said to Richard that if the outcome of my disease was not a success and the worst happened to me, I wanted him to carry out my wishes. One of them was that I would like to donate my organs to medical research. Richard said, "Oh, be sure and leave them your brain then, as it's hardly been used!"

I remembered that I received an invitation from a local crematorium for a social wine and cheese party in order to discuss future designs in urns, where I'd like to be scattered, and that sort of thing. Believe it or not, this was the same day I was diagnosed with cancer! They could not have known how bad their timing was. I told my loved ones, "I don't care what you do with me, ultimately; just don't tell me what it will be beforehand."

Future Ambitions after Recovery

I have lots of plans when I start feeling a bit better. One of them is that I would love to meet Oprah one day. Actually, I've wanted to for quite a while. Oprah was born the same year as I was, and look what she's achieved compared to me! Anyway, she has inspired not only me but also a great number of people. She is a wonderful example of what my husband and I have learned and experienced by living in the United States for twenty-five years as guests of this country.

For me, she exemplifies the idea that if you have a talent—and we all do, in some form or another—work hard at it, and never give up; you can achieve whatever you wish in life. So I just wanted to say thank you to Oprah, and thank you, America, for putting up with us Brits...so far, at least.

Oh, and before I forget—again—the other person whom I want to meet is Adele. Despite her unearthly, beautiful singing voice, her monumental talent, and her rise to stardom at a very young age, she is—and always will be—herself. "What you see is what you get," basically. I recently read a *Time* magazine article about her in my plastic surgeon's office, but I couldn't concentrate while reading it, of course. Yet in my foggy state, I understood that she's adored by all of us, and rightly so.

I love the fact that she openly admits that she came from humble beginnings. She doesn't seem to get fazed by any of the obvious media attention, because of her start in life. When interviewed, she is completely honest. She is also very funny. I loved watching the Carpool Karaoke with James Corden; it was just wonderful. Anyway, I could write a book...oh wait, I am. Richard said that there are two hopes of meeting these two celebrities...Bob and no—but you'll only get that one if you're in your dotage and probably not expected to last through the night. To translate for younger readers, Richard meant Bob Hope and no hope!

Family and friends

There are people in our lives who are angels masquerading as people on earth, and I know lots of them. My best friend—my husband, Richard—is one of them. He has given me lots of love and support, as he always does, which has helped me cope while going through this ordeal. He is a fantastic nurse, and he reminded me constantly to do all the things I was supposed to in order to recover quickly and get back to some sort of normality. He was also a constant source of kindness, understanding, and everything your spouse should be in your time of need. He has also had to endure the extremes of emotions that one experiences with this disease, like being overly angry about a situation you would normally shrug off or laughing uproariously about something that is only mildly amusing in reality. Truthfully, you really are "away with the fairies" for quite a few weeks. His wicked sense of humor kept us going, too, and he was a source of light relief on many a hospital visit or doctor's appointment. If only briefly, he definitely took my mind off what was happening to me. So Richard, full marks—you passed the "husband exam" with flying colors.

My dearest friend, Linda Lillmars, is another one of these angels. Strangely enough, Linda has been with me whenever something awful has happened in my life and has gently looked after me in her quiet, nurturing way when I needed a mother figure. I remember shortly after my surgery, I was having a really bad pain day, and I had to go back to bed in the middle of the day, which isn't like me. I was curled up in the fetal position in bed with my head buried in the pillow, crying with pain. I managed to call Linda in Alaska, and she talked me through the pain, and I have no idea to this day how long a time it was. The pain gradually started to wear off, and it was my Linda, being my own special angel again, doing what she does, as always. Most of the wonderful friends I have, if I called them at three o'clock in the morning and asked them to come and help, they'd be there in a flash with no questions asked.

I have received cards, flowers, messages, and many kindnesses from all our friends, and we are so very touched by this. It has been quite overwhelming, actually, and very humbling. This also aids in a quicker recovery, so again, Richard and I thank everyone for their fabulous friendship and support.

My family has been wonderful, and although they all live in the UK, I have had constant kind notes and phone calls and the knowledge that they were thinking of me and sending their love. The world has become much smaller because of Skype and FaceTime, which is great. I can now see my loved ones as if they're in the same room as me, which is also great.

Medical staff

I would like to thank the wonderful staff at Methodist West Breast Care Center. From the ladies who checked me in to the radiographers, the radiologist, and all the staff—thank you so very much. The staff were so kind to me in a very frightening situation, which I really appreciated. There were four ladies in the room when I had my biopsy; one held my hand, another comforted me, and they were so gentle and efficient. Their facility is brand new and very well equipped with everything a patient might need, from state-of-the-art technology and a beautiful waiting area to warmed gowns to change into while waiting for your mammogram. Thank you, everyone.

I would like to thank my plastic surgeon, Dr. Warren Ellsworth IV; his nurse, Ally Verheul, RN; his PA, Amanda Stewart; and his entire team at Methodist West Hospital. My care was excellent in every respect. They explained everything to me so well, and I knew I was receiving first-class treatment—thank you. They were also very patient with me and my sense of humor, and the fact that sometimes I was a little confused, to put it mildly. Thank you again.

Thank you to the world-class team at The University of Texas, MD Anderson Cancer Center: my radiation oncologist, Dr. Elizabeth Bloom; her nurse, Kimberly Yerrow, RN; and all her wonderful staff in Katy. I especially want to thank the ladies who looked after me in the radiation room—the radiation therapists, Susan Bullion, RTT, and Andrea Machuca, RTT. Seeing them every single day for four weeks in an intimate situation made us very close, and we became friends. I looked forward to seeing them every day, and we would enjoy ourselves despite the somewhat harrowing circumstances. Again, I knew I was in good hands, and they were very kind and patient with me; they made me as comfortable as possible at each session. Thank you so much to everyone.

Thank you to my oncology surgeon, Dr. Jessica Suarez-Colen, and her staff at the Memorial City location. Again, I received the finest care from everyone. Thank you so much.

Last, but not least, I would like to thank my oncologist, Dr. Nikesh Jasani, and his staff at the Katy location. I cannot thank everyone enough for my care, for which my husband, Richard, and I are eternally grateful.

I am very fortunate to have had the finest possible care for my cancer. I could not live in a better place than Houston while suffering from any type of cancer with MD Anderson taking care of me. People fly here from all over the world for treatment and to be cared for by this elite team of medical professionals. So, think positive thoughts and do what they tell you to do in order to help yourself. Hopefully, things will go well for you in your recovery. I believe that Shakespeare once wrote, "Brevity is the soul of wit," so I'll shut up now.

The End